Blood sugar resolution: The Life-Changing Impact of Blood Sugar Balancing

by

Kevin T. McHugh

Table of contents

Introduction

Blood glucose or blood sugar is what it's called as it goes via your bloodstream to your cells. Insulin is a hormone that transports glucose from the bloodstream into cells for energy and storage.

Diabetes patients have higher-than-normal glucose levels in their blood. They either don't have enough insulin, or their cells don't respond to insulin as well as they should.

Long-term high blood glucose levels can harm your kidneys, eyes, and other organs.

Chapter 1

What is glucose

Glucose is the primary type of sugar in the blood and is the major energy source for the body's cells. The body can create glucose from other substances or obtain it from our food. The bloodstream carries glucose to the cells. The hormone insulin is one of many that regulates blood glucose levels. Glucose may also be referred to as blood sugar. The body's internal processes depend on glucose to function properly. It often goes unnoticed when our glucose levels are at their ideal ranges. However, you'll see the unfavorable impact it has on people when they depart from the advised limits. Everyday functioning. So what is glucose, exactly? It's the simplest monosaccharide, having only one type of sugar. It has one sugar.

Thus this indicates. It's not by itself. Galactose, ribose, and fructose are examples of additional monosaccharides. Glucose is one of the body's preferred fuels, along with fat. Fuel sources in the form of sugars. Bread, fruits, vegetables, and dairy products all contain glucose.

To produce the energy that keeps you alive, you need food. While glucose is necessary, like with many things, it's best in moderation. Glucose levels that are unhealthy or out of control can have permanent and severe effects.

Importance of glucose to the body

It serves as brain fuel: Usually, the brain gets all of its energy almost solely from glucose. The brain needs a steady supply of glucose due to its high energy requirements and inability to retain it. The body has several defenses against hypoglycemia or a severe drop in blood sugar levels.

But if there is such a dip, the brain can start to malfunction. Common brain-related hypoglycemia symptoms include headache, dizziness, disorientation, lack of focus, anxiety, irritability, restlessness, slurred speech, and poor coordination. Seizures and coma are possible outcomes of a quick, dramatic drop in blood glucose.

Good For Muscles: Depending on sex, age, and fitness level, the skeletal muscles typically make up between 30 and 40 percent of the total body weight. During the activity, the skeletal muscles need a lot of glucose. Skeletal muscles store blood sugar in the form of glycogen, which is readily broken down to provide glucose during physical activity, in contrast to the brain. Additionally, muscle tissue typically absorbs enormous amounts of glucose through physical exertion from the blood. Even though skeletal muscles can use molecules generated from fat as an energy source, the depletion of glucose reserves during prolonged activity can cause rapid exhaustion, also known as bonking or hitting the wall.

Fuel for Other Tissues and Organs: The body's numerous organs and tissues can use a variety of fuels. Some other significant organs and tissues, besides the brain and skeletal muscles, depend on glucose as their main or only fuel source. Examples include the red and white blood cells as well as the cornea, lens, and retina of the eyes. It's interesting to note that although the small intestine's/*-cells are in charge of absorbing glucose from food and transferring it to the bloodstream they mostly use glutamine as a fuel source. This frees up more glucose for other tissues and organs that depend on sugar more.

Structural Roles: The human body uses glucose and other chemicals to create other crucial structural components in addition to its function in energy production. One such instance is the glycoprotein collagen, which has a protein backbone and simple carbohydrates like glucose. Skin, muscles, bones, and other human tissues contain collagen, an important structural component. Other glycoproteins significantly influence the growth and upkeep of the body's nerves. Glycolipids, made up of fat and sugar building blocks, are essential parts of the membranes that envelop and support each of the body's cells.

What is Hypoglycemia

If you have hypoglycemia, your blood sugar (glucose) level is below the normal range. Your body uses glucose as its primary energy source.Hypoglycemia and diabetes management frequently go hand in hand.

Low blood sugar can, however, occur in persons without diabetes due to various diseases and other medications, many of which are uncommon. Treating hypoglycemia is necessary. A fasting blood sugar reading of 70 mg/dL, or 3.9 mmol/L, or lower should be a warning sign for hypoglycemia in many people. Your figures, however, might be different. Inquire with your doctor. The goal of treatment is to lower your blood sugar as rapidly as possible, either with a high-sugar meal or beverage or by taking medication. It is necessary to determine and address the cause of hypoglycemia for long-term treatment.

Symptoms

Hypoglycemia symptoms and indicators can appear if blood sugar levels go too low and include:

- appearing pale
- Shakiness
- Sweating
- Headache

- Lips, tongue, or cheek tingling or numbness

Signs and symptoms of hypoglycemia can include:

Unusual behavior, confusion, or both, such as the

inability to carry out daily chores Unsteady speech

fuzziness or tunnel vision nightmares when sleeping

Extreme hypoglycemia may result in:

Unresponsiveness (loss of consciousness)

Seizures

Whenever to visit a doctor, Immediately seek medical attention if You might have signs of hypoglycemia, but you don't have diabetes. You have diabetes, and nothing seems to work despite trying to manage your hypoglycemia by drinking juice or regular (not diet) soft drinks, eating candy, or taking glucose tablets. If you have diabetes or a history of hypoglycemia and you experience severe hypoglycemia symptoms or become unconscious, you should seek emergency medical attention.

Cause OF Hypoglycemia

You have hypoglycemia when your blood sugar (glucose) level drops too low for normal bodily functions to continue. This may occur for several reasons. Low blood sugar is most frequently caused by a side effect of diabetes treatments.

Chapter 2

Blood sugar control

Your body converts food into glucose when you eat. Insulin, a hormone made by the pancreas, aids in the entry of glucose, the body's primary energy source, into the cells. Insulin enables glucose to enter the cells and supply the energy required by your cells. Your muscles and liver both contain glycogen, which is a sort of extra glucose storage. You will cease manufacturing insulin when you haven't eaten in several hours, and your blood sugar level falls. The pancreatic hormone glucagon instructs your liver to release glucose into your bloodstream by dissolving the glycogen that has been stored in your body.

Until you eat again, this keeps your blood sugar levels within a normal range. Glucose can also be produced by your body. Your kidneys and liver both play a significant role in this process. The body can break down fat reserves and utilize the byproducts of fat breakdown as an alternate fuel during extended fasting.

Potential causes involving diabetes

If you have diabetes, you may not produce insulin (type 1 diabetes), or you may respond to insulin less favorably (type 2 diabetes). As a result, blood glucose levels increase and occasionally rise to dangerously high levels.

You might use insulin or other blood sugarlowering drugs to solve this issue. However, taking too much insulin or other diabetic drugs might result in hypoglycemia, which is when your blood sugar level drops too low. In addition, hypoglycemia might happen if you exercise more than normal or eat less than usual after taking your daily dose of diabetic medication.

Potential causes without diabetes

People without diabetes are substantially less likely to experience hypoglycemia. Medicines can be one of the causes. Accidentally ingesting someone else's oral diabetic medicine can result in hypoglycemia. Other drugs have the potential to cause hypoglycemia, particularly in young patients or those with kidney disease. One illustration is the malaria drug quinine (Qualaquin). Excessive alcohol consumption Drinking excessively without eating can prevent the liver from releasing glucose into the bloodstream from its glycogen stores. The result may be hypoglycemia.

A few serious illnesses. Hypoglycemia can be brought on by severe infections, kidney disease, advanced heart disease, and liver diseases such as severe cirrhosis or hepatitis. Additionally, kidney problems can prevent your body from adequately eliminating drugs. An accumulation of drugs that lower blood sugar levels may have an impact on glucose levels.

Prolonged starvation Malnutrition and famine can cause hypoglycemia because when you don't eat enough, your body uses up the glycogen stores it requires to produce glucose. One condition that can result in hypoglycemia and long-term malnutrition is an eating disorder termed anorexia nervosa. A surplus of insulin you can develop hypoglycemia if your pancreas produces too much insulin due to a rare pancreatic tumor called an insulinoma. A surplus of insulin-like molecules can also be produced as a result of other cancers. The pancreas' peculiar cells can cause excessive insulin release, which leads to hypoglycemia.Hormonal imbalances. Specific diseases of the pituitary and adrenal glands may cause insufficient levels of certain hormones that control glucose synthesis or metabolism.

If a child has too little growth hormone, they may have hypoglycemia. A surplus of insulin. You can develop hypoglycemia if your pancreas produces too much insulin due to a rare pancreatic tumor called an insulinoma.

Hypoglycemia following a meal

Usually, but not always, hypoglycemia happens after not eating. After particular meals, hypoglycemic symptoms can appear, but it is unclear why.

Reactive hypoglycemia, also known as postprandial hypoglycemia, can happen in patients who have undergone procedures that alter the stomach's normal function. Although stomach bypass surgery is the procedure most frequently linked to this, it can also happen to patients who have had other surgeries.

Complications

Hypoglycemia left untreated might result in:

Seizure, Coma and Death

Hypoglycemia may also result in:

- Falling

- Feelingweek

- Injuries

- collisions

Dementia risk is higher in older adults

Ignorance of Hypoglycemia

Hypoglycemia unawareness can develop over time as a result of recurrent hypoglycemic episodes. Low blood sugar warning signs and symptoms like trembling or irregular heartbeats are no longer produced by the body or brain (palpitations). The possibility of severe, potentially fatal hypoglycemia rises when this occurs.

Your healthcare practitioner may change your therapy, raise your blood sugar level objectives, and suggest blood glucose awareness training if you have diabetes, recurrent hypoglycemia, and hypoglycemia unawareness. Some patients with hypoglycemia unawareness can use a continuous glucose monitor (CGM). Your blood sugar can be too low, and the device can warn you of it.

Chapter 3

Source of Glucose

The most prevalent monosaccharide in nature is glucose. It is produced by photosynthesis in plants. Chains of linked glucose are stored by some plants. Starch is the name for these chains. Foods that frequently contain starch include corn, potatoes, rice, and wheat. From these whole food sources, starch is professionally separated to create dextrose, glucose, maltodextrins, polyols, and high fructose corn syrup, which are then used as ingredients to create a variety of foods, drinks, dressings, and sauces.

Some foods naturally include glucose monosaccharides; however not part of the starch component. Honey and dried fruits, including dates, apricots, raisins, currants, cranberries, prunes, and figs, are the two sources of glucose monosaccharides in the highest concentration in whole foods.

How can plants derive glucose?

Plants absorb water (H_2O) and carbon dioxide (CO_2) from the soil and atmosphere during photosynthesis. Water is oxidized, which means it loses electrons, while carbon dioxide is reduced, which means it receives electrons inside the plant cell.

Water is converted into oxygen and carbon dioxide into glucose as a result. After storing energy within the glucose molecules, the plant releases the oxygen back into the atmosphere.

Examples of foods high in glucose

Tomato Canned Nothing on your pantry shelf is more practical than a can of tomato sauce. 6.1 grams of glucose and a great amount of potassium, iron, and vitamin C are both found in one cup of canned tomato puree. Try these hearty (tomato sauce-based, non-noodle) meals instead of sticking to just pasta. When you're in the mood for a pulled pork sandwich, jackfruit is a got-to-meat substitute. Jackfruit slices contain 15.6 grams of glucose per cup. This fruit is a high source of vitamin C, magnesium, and potassium and has a stringy texture akin to pulled meat.

Jackfruit contains fewer than 3 grams of protein per cup, which is a low amount compared to many other plant-based meat alternatives.

Cherries, the smallest stone fruit, contain 10.1 grams of glucose per cup. According to a review published in Nutrients in March 2018, cherries are high in polyphenols, a naturally occurring plant component that studies have linked to a lower risk for metabolic syndrome, diabetes, and nonalcoholic fatty liver disease (NAFLD), and heart disease.

Chapter 4

Importance of measuring blood glucose levels

Measurement of blood glucose levels is essential. Monitoring your blood sugar levels can help you figure out whether you are hitting your glucose goals, which can help you avoid long-term diabetic issues and lessen the unpleasant effects of high and low blood sugar. The figures are neither excellent nor negative and are crucial to keeping in mind. They are only tools for learning what practical and pinpointing areas for development in your diabetes treatment are.

Because A1C tests are only performed every 3-6 months and only provide an average, blood sugar monitoring is crucial. Even with an A1C in the target range, a person may nevertheless experience frequent high and low blood sugar readings.The need and effectiveness of blood sugar monitoring. You and your medical team should decide how frequently you should monitor your blood sugar. In general, patients with type 1 diabetes who use an insulin pump, take numerous daily insulin injections, or any of these should check their blood sugar more regularly.

Anytime they suspect low blood sugar, including after treating low blood sugar, until blood sugar has returned to 70mg/dL or higher, they should check their blood sugar level. This includes before all meals and snacks, at bedtime, before exercising, and before engaging in potentially dangerous activities like driving. This can be done manually or automatically with continuous glucose monitoring, ranging from six to ten times each day (CGM). When modifying the diet plan, physical exercise or medications for patients with type 2 diabetes who don't take insulin or only take it once a day, monitoring blood sugar levels can be helpful.

A person with type 2 diabetes, for instance, might check once or twice day, alternating between before meals and before bed, but some people prefer to check more frequently. Checking blood sugar levels before meals to evaluate if you are hitting your goals is one technique for glucose monitoring. You can check your blood sugar before a meal and again within 1-2 hours after it to see how you're doing once readings before a meal are at the target level. Without additionally taking some sort of action, simply gathering data is useless.

To understand how to respond and increase the amount of time you spend in the target range, it is crucial to discuss the information with your healthcare team and to schedule regular meetings with a diabetes care and education specialist.

How Your Body Makes Glucose

It primarily originates from foods high in carbs, such as fruit, bread, and potatoes. Food moves from your mouth to your stomach via your esophagus while you eat. It is reduced to tiny fragments by acids and enzymes there. This causes the release of glucose. It goes into your intestines, where it's absorbed. From there, it passes into your bloodstream. Once in the blood, insulin helps glucose get to your cells.

Chapter 5

Factors that affects blood sugar

There are 42 factors known to affect blood sugar levels, and different persons may react differently to these factors. For instance, some people may genuinely experience an increase in blood sugar after drinking a cup

of black coffee without any sugar or milk, while others may not. Check your blood sugar levels before, during, and after ingestion to learn how you react differently. To directly calculate the effects, a continuous glucose monitor (CGM) could be worn as an alternative. Physical exercise is another illustration. Light activity, such as walking, lowers blood sugar levels for many people, while it has little effect on others. High-intensity exercise like running can cause some people's blood sugar to go down, but for some, it will actually go up.

The time of day, level of fitness and training, and the amount of sleep you got the night before can all play a role in this. Tracking the data from blood sugar monitoring (BGM) is a valuable way to learn about yourself.

Symptoms of low blood sugar

When a person produces too much insulin or gets too much medication, it can cause low blood sugar. Blood sugar between 54-69mg/dL is considered level hypoglycemia.

Typical symptoms of low blood sugar include:

Dizziness

Irregular or fast heartbeat

Hunger

Sweating

Anxiety

Irritability

Shakiness

Some people may feel symptoms above 70mg/dL, while others don't feel symptoms until levels are even lower. Level 2 hypoglycemia is considered a blood sugar under 54mg/dL. This can lead to more severe symptoms such as confusion, abnormal behavior, and blurred vision because, at this point, the brain may not be getting enough glucose to function. When glucose gets too low, this can lead to a person falling, having seizures, or passing out.

Level 3 hypoglycemia is when a person can't think clearly or may have passed out and needed the assistance of another person. This response is not defined by a specific glucose value. When a person does not get enough insulin or medication to meet their body's demands, it can lead to high blood sugar or hyperglycemia. There are many causes of hyperglycemia, including untreated diabetes, not getting enough medication, eating too many carbohydrates, being less physically active, having excess weight, and genetic factors.

Typical symptoms of high blood sugar include:

- Extreme thirst
- The need to urinate often
- Blurry vision
- Increased hunger
- Feeling tired and weak
- Headache

Other symptoms can be severe and could include vomiting, confusion, shortness of breath, and even coma. Some symptoms of low and high blood sugar can be similar, like blurred vision and drowsiness. Therefore, it is important to check blood sugar before treating it.

Symptoms of high blood sugar

When a person does not get enough insulin or medication to meet their body's demands, it can lead to high blood sugar or hyperglycemia. There are many causes of hyperglycemia, including untreated diabetes, not getting enough medication, eating too many carbohydrates, being less physically active, having excess weight, and genetic factors

Other symptoms can be severe and could include vomiting, confusion, shortness of breath, and even coma. Some symptoms of low blood sugar and high blood sugar can be similar, like blurred vision and drowsiness. Therefore, it is important to check blood sugar before treatment.

Treatment of low and high blood sugar

Low blood sugar can be treated with a fast-acting carbohydrate such as juice, regular soda, hard candies (not chocolate), or glucose tablets. People often ask, why not chocolate? This is because it contains fat, and fat will make the carbohydrate slower to absorb, taking blood sugar longer to recover. It typically takes 15 minutes for blood sugar to rise. If a person is using insulin, it's important not to take any insulin with the glucose treatment. If, after checking blood sugar again in 15 minutes, it's still below 70mg/dL, the glucose intake can be repeated.

Once blood sugar is above 70mg/dL, a person should continue to eat a complete meal or snack that includes protein, such as half a sandwich or peanut butter and crackers. If a person is passed out or unable to consume food or liquids, glucagon can be used as an emergency treatment. Glucagon is available as either an injection or nasal powder. Every person with diabetes at risk of low blood sugar should have a prescription for glucagon.

1. Exercise regularly

Regular exercise can help you reach and maintain a moderate weight and increase insulin sensitivity. Increased insulin sensitivity means your cells can more effectively use the available sugar in your bloodstream. Exercise also helps your muscles use blood sugar for energy and muscle contraction. If you have problems with blood sugar management, consider routinely checking your levels before and after exercising.

This will help you learn how you respond to different activities and keep your blood sugar levels from getting too high or low. What's more, researchers recommend making so-called "exercise snacks" to lower blood sugar and prevent the damage that sitting all day can cause. Exercise snacks simply mean that you break up your sitting time every 30 minutes for just a few minutes throughout the day.

Some of the recommended exercises include light walking or simple resistance exercises like squats or leg raises.

2. Manage your carb intake

Your blood sugar levels are significantly impacted by the number of carbohydrates you consume. Carbs are converted by your body into sugars, primarily glucose. Insulin then assists your body in using and storing it for energy. This process breaks down, and blood glucose levels can increase when you consume too many carbohydrates or have issues with insulin function. Due to this, the American Diabetes Association (ADA) advises patients with diabetes to control their carb intake by measuring their intake and understanding how many they require.

According to some research, doing this will help you properly plan your meals, which can further enhance blood sugar control.

A low-carb diet helps lower blood sugar levels and prevent blood sugar spikes, according to numerous research. It's important to note that lowcarb diets and no-carb diets are not the same. You can still eat some carbs when monitoring your blood sugar. However, prioritizing whole grains over processed ones and refined carbs provides more excellent nutritional value while helping decrease your blood sugar levels

3. Eat more fiber

Fiber slows carb digestion and sugar absorption, promoting a more gradual rise in blood sugar levels. There are two types of fiber— insoluble and soluble. While both are important, soluble fiber has been shown to improve blood sugar management, while insoluble fiber hasn't been shown to have this effect. A high-fiber diet can improve your body's ability to regulate blood sugar and minimize blood sugar lows.

4. 4 Aim for low-glycemic-index foods.

The glycemic index (GI) gauges how quickly your body consumes carbohydrates and how quickly they break down after digestion. The rate at which your blood sugar levels rise is impacted by this. Foods are classified as low, medium, or high GI according to the GI, which rates them from 0 to 100. The ranking of low GI meals is 55 or lower. The quantity and kind of carbohydrates you consume both affect how a portion of food affects your blood sugar levels. Particularly, eating low GI meals has been demonstrated to lower blood sugar levels in diabetics.

Some examples of foods with a low to moderate GI include: Bulgur barley unsweetened Greek yogurt

- oats
- beans
- lentils
- legumes

Furthermore, adding protein or healthy fats helps minimize blood sugar spikes after a meal

5. Try to manage your stress levels

Stress can affect your blood sugar levels. When stressed, your body secretes hormones called glucagon and cortisol, which cause blood sugar levels to rise. One study including a group of students showed that exercise, relaxation, and meditation significantly reduced stress and lowered blood sugar levels Exercises and relaxation methods like yoga and mindfulness-based stress reduction may also help correct insulin secretion problems among people with chronic diabetes

6. Monitor your blood sugar levels

Monitoring blood glucose levels can help you better manage them. You can do so at home using a portable blood glucose meter, which is known as a glucometer. You can discuss this option with your doctor. Keeping track allows you to determine whether you need to adjust your meals or medications. It also helps you learn how your body reacts to certain foods. Try measuring your levels regularly every day and keeping track of the numbers in a log. Also, it may be more helpful to track your blood sugar in pairs — for example, before and after exercise or before and 2 hours after a meal.

This can show you whether you need to make small changes to a meal if it spikes your blood sugar rather than avoiding your favorite meals altogether. Some adjustments include swapping a starchy side for non-starchy veggies or limiting them to a handful.

Conclusion

Glucose is used as the body's main energy source. When the level of glucose in your blood is too high or low, various health problems can occur. If this is left untreated, it can affect various parts of the body, from the eyes to the kidneys. If your blood sugar levels fall outside of the normal range, contact your healthcare provider.

Despite the widespread use of herbs and medicinal plants, the effectiveness of using phytochemicals to treat diabetes has not been supported by scientific evidence that may warrant their replacement with the existing medication. The high quantity of flavonoids in citrus species, particularly naringenin, narirutin, rutin, and vimentin-2, has some promise for the treatment of diabetes, albeit no one species is exactly comparable to human diabetes. Furthermore, the other common SGLT2 inhibitors shared similar skeletal architectures with citrus backbones.

Each model serves as a crucial tool for researching treatments as Type 2 diabetes in humans has progressed.

.3